The Magic & Mystery of Marijuana

Understanding The Cannabis Plant

By
Vern Kirby

Copyrighted Material

Copyright © 2022 -Vern Kirby

All Rights Reserved

No part of this publication may be reproduced, stored in a retrieval system, or transmitted in any form or means, electronic, mechanical photocopying, recording or otherwise, without the proper written consent of the copyright holder, except for a brief quotation used in a review.

Published By:

Vern Kirby

Houston, Texas

First Edition

Legal Disclaimer

This book is written for the sole purpose of providing information to the readers. The publisher and author, or anyone else associated with the production of this book, do not advocate breaking or violating any federal, state, or other local laws. However, we strongly support the passage of fair marijuana and cannabis legislation.

It should also be noted that the legal aspects of growing, and the consumption of marijuana vary in different countries; hence, readers are advised to use their own discretion and abide by the rules of the country.

Also, this book is not intended to be a substitute for the medical advice of doctors. The readers are advised to consult a physician in matters related to his/her health relating to the use of cannabis or marijuana.

Ecclesiastes 3:1

To everything there is a season, and a time for every purpose under the heaven

Table Of Contents

Introduction	7
History Of Cannabis	11
Endocannaboid System	17
Addiction & Withdrawal	23
Prohibition, Prisons & FDA	33
Industrial Hemp & Reefer Madness	41
CBD Products	55
Restoration Of Body	65
My Story	69
Conclusion	95

Published and copyrighted in 2022

By Vern Kirby

Introduction

At age 78, I made the decision to stop smoking marijuana. I also plan to stop taking Cannabidiol (CBD) products. After using marijuana for over 50 years and realizing many benefits from its use, I have made this decision based on some unexplained causes of symptoms that I have experienced over the last few years. I am extremely healthy, and this opinion is shared by my doctors. I take no prescription medications for chronic conditions; however, I have experienced several symptoms that no doctor has been able to explain. My decision to stop using cannabis is based on the possibility that these symptoms are a side effect of cannabis use. The only way to determine this is by stopping the use of it.

Today, marijuana is available legally to over 60% of the United States population by state governments. Yet it remains illegally federally available as a Schedule One drug. Because of the federal Schedule One classification, little research has been done on the properties of cannabis and its effect on our bodies. However, industrial hemp, which was previously also classified as a Schedule One drug, has been removed as a Schedule One drug in recent legislation. Industrial hemp is now legal to grow across the United States, subject to state and local laws. Since Industrial Hemp is low in Tetrahydrocannabinol (THC) and high in CBD content, one of the first markets for this new farming opportunity is CBD products. I have used CBD for about six years.

The official name for both marijuana and hemp today is cannabis. Limited research today has determined that our bodies have a system called the endocannabinoid system, which affects virtually every cell in our bodies. The legal distinction between the legal use of hemp and the legal use of marijuana is determined by the content of the cannabinoids within the plant. The two used for this are THC and CBD. Since THC is the element which produces psychotropic effects that get you high, it has stricter requirements by the government. Since CBD does not produce the level of intoxication of THC, it is deemed legal for industrial use.

Both THC and CBD have been determined to have beneficial properties for health and medicinal purposes. Industrial hemp has many uses not related to our bodies but instead for industrial use such as papers, fuels, cloth, and thousands of other products. While some research on our endocannabinoid system has identified the effects of THC and CBD, there are about 100 other cannabinoids in our bodies that are yet unexplained. This fact is the reason I have made my decision. I feel some conditions in my body may be side effects of the presence of some of these as well.

I was born in 1943, just a few years after our government launched a campaign called "reefer madness." I started using marijuana when I was 28 years old. The mindset of society at that time was that marijuana was a dangerous drug outlawed and punishable as a felony. For that reason, my early use was both very private, and I had no discussion with any doctor about it. As time passed, more, people began to use marijuana and the claims of the government's reefer madness program have been discredited.

In recent years, I have been able to discuss my use with doctors and it is obvious that many of the health benefits I enjoy may be the result of this use. I consider myself to be a law-abiding citizen and have never been arrested for any drug violations, but I know people who have. I feel legalization is overdue. The damage from marijuana has been more from the fact that it has been illegal rather than from the drug itself. In fact, I am not sure if it should even be classified as a drug, but a food supplement.

Cannabis has a history that dates back 6000 years or more B.C. It has been prohibited for use in the United States legally for about 75 years. It remains a Schedule One drug federally approved today.

As I began this project, I have been free from marijuana and cannabidiol (CBD) use for about four weeks. I understand that it may take several months for my body to return to a completely natural state. My intention is to share my understanding of the history of cannabis, share more details of my story with addiction and my relationship with God. I will outline where we stand today.

Hopefully, this will enable people to have a better understanding of the benefits of marijuana use, as well is the importance of its use in moderation. Not only should cannabis be legalized, but research should also be put in place to help understand the full impact it can have on society.

There are many benefits as a nutritional supplement, with industrial products and medicines. It is in direct competition with many pharmaceutical products, petroleum products and an ideal commodity for the manufacturer of paper, cloth, and many other products. The Internet provides an abundance of information, some of which is contradictory. The things I say here are my own opinions based on 50 years of use, internet research, and prayer with God. The following pages will outline my life with addiction, my understanding of cannabis, and my relationship with God.

Chapter One

History of Cannabis

Once upon a time, there was a plant called cannabis. Since as far back as 10,000 years ago, it was one of the first crops grown when farming began. Hemp, a variety of the cannabis plants, has consistently been used in places like ancient China to create clothing, paper, and rope. Hemp was and still is non- psychoactive, which means it does not affect the mind or mental processes because its THC levels are so low. In other words, smoking it will not get you high.

The first recorded use of cannabis as a medicine was not until approximately 2737 B.C. Emperor Shenlong of China used the plant as medicine for things like gout, malaria, and poor memory. Throughout the next 3000 years, cannabis was used for many medicinal purposes. Slowly, it spread throughout Asia and into Europe. The Chinese mixed it into food. In ancient India, they mixed it into a drink called bang. In Greece, cannabis seeds have been consumed recreationally. A Chinese doctor used cannabis to relieve pain for patients undergoing surgery. He would grind it and mix it with wine. During the

Middle Ages, cannabis was popular in the Middle East. Muslims there were not supposed to drink wine, but nobody said they could not smoke grass. That is what they did. They called it hashish. Christopher Columbus brought rope made from hemp on his first voyage to the new world in 1492. The French and British had their colonists grow cannabis in the new world during the 1600s.

Cannabis grew even more popular and became a major thing to trade between South and Central Asia in the 1700s. Doctors everywhere recommended cannabis as a medicine. The Irish doctor William O'Shaughnessy helped popularize its medical use for pain treatment.

In 1798, Napoleon learned that many of his soldiers had started smoking cannabis while in Egypt. They brought the habit back with them to France. In response, he outlawed the plant.

Still, cannabis remained popular in the 1800s. Cannabis plantations were scattered around the United States. Doctors regularly prescribed it and it was easy to buy in general stores. People were trained for the cultivation and use of cannabis all around the world, and its use dramatically increased by the end of the 1800s.

Attitudes toward cannabis started to change near the end of the 1880s. A growing number of people were freaking out about drugs in general, as alcoholism and opium addiction were dramatically on the rise.

The British led the charge. They passed the first modern log of certain dangerous drugs. In 1868, many soon began to believe that cannabis use caused mental illness. In 1893, the British government became concerned with cannabis use in India, which they controlled at the time. They issued a study called the Indian Hemp Drugs Commission, which found that moderate cannabis use was fine and that it did not make people go crazy.

In the United States, the Progressive Era swept the country, and many progressives called for stricter regulations against potentially harmful drugs. In 1906, the US government passed the Pure Food and Drug Act, which said cannabis was dangerous and required it be labeled before being sold.

In 1913, California became the first state to ban growing cannabis. In 1914, the Harrison Narcotics Tax Act officially made drug use a crime for the first time. Meanwhile, cannabis had become more known as a recreational drug as opposed to a medicinal one. More people began to smoke it in cigarettes or pipes.

Many Mexicans smoked it. After millions of illegal Mexican immigrants flooded into the United States, due to the Mexican Revolution, they brought the habit with them. Mexicans call cannabis marijuana. Mexicans became strongly associated with smoking cannabis. Americans were xenophobic of Mexicans, anyway, and became more afraid of cannabis due to the association.

In 1928, the United Kingdom prohibited cannabis. By the early 1930s, the world was going through the Great Depression and eagerly looking for something or someone to blame for its devastation. Mexican immigrants became scapegoats. One man is responsible for cannabis becoming illegal, more so than any other person in history. That man is Harry J. Anslinger. He was the first commissioner of the Federal Bureau of Narcotics and launched a relentless campaign against cannabis use.

Testifying before Congress to get them to make the plant illegal, the following are actual quotes from Harry J. Anslinger. "There are 100,000 total marijuana smokers in the US, and most are Negroes, Hispanics, Filipinos and entertainers." Their satanic music, jazz and swing resulted from marijuana usage. This marijuana causes white women to seek sexual relations with Negroes, entertainers, and any others." "Reefer makes darkies think they're as good as white men." "Marijuana is the most violent drug in the history of mankind." Notice how he described cannabis as marijuana, so making it sound, more foreign, and associated with immigrants from Mexico. From this point forward, marijuana became the most common way of referring to the drug.

Anslinger never said much about marijuana when alcohol was still illegal. In 1936, with the help of Anslinger, the film "Reefer Madness" showed a false story of good people getting violent and going crazy due to using marijuana.

Eventually, millions saw anti-marijuana propaganda. All of this helped lead the United States Congress to pass the Marijuana Tax Act of 1937, which regulated marijuana by requiring those that sold it to pay an exceedingly high tax. The media barely paid attention and few debated the law; in fact, most approved the law even though they know little about marijuana.

The only one to speak out against the bill in the hearings before it passed was William Woodward, a representative for the American Medical Association. He said they knew of no evidence that marijuana was dangerous and that outlawing it loses sight of the fact that future investigation and research may show that there are substantial medical uses for cannabis.

Congress ignored Woodward and passed the law, anyway. Suddenly, even doctors were afraid of marijuana. On October 2nd, 1937, Samuel Caldwell became the first person in American history arrested for selling it. By this time, Canada and China had also outlawed marijuana and the culture around the world had changed.

Although in places like the Middle East, Northern Africa and India, people still could consume it. By this time, the United States was the top dog in the world and therefore influenced laws related to marijuana.

The Prohibition we know today began with "Reefer Madness," a false narrative that spread to other countries. Prohibition and "Reefer Madness" are described in a later chapter.

Chapter Two

The Endocannabinoid System

The endocannabinoid system (ECS) plays critical roles in many biological processes, ranging from pain sensitivity to immune function. Everything we know about this elaborate system has been discovered within the last 50 years.

Understanding began with a simple question about the medicinal properties of the plant known as cannabis. Indigenous to Eastern Asia with records of therapeutic and recreational use dating back more than 45 centuries.

While the clinical effects of cannabis on basic body functions were well known, the chemical constituent responsible for its actions remained a mystery until 1964.

An Israeli chemist Amahle visually identified and isolated D9-tetrahydrocannabinol or THC for the first time. Further exploration of how THC and other fighter cannabinoids worked was hindered by the limited technologies available to molecular biologists and chemists at the time.

It wasn't until 1988, when THC was found to bind to a receptor, which is abundantly expressed in the brain, particularly in regions responsible for cognition emotions, appetite, and motor coordination. THC's ability to attach to receptors in the brain explained many of its psychotropic effects, but it couldn't explain its peripheral actions.

In 1993, a second cannabinoids receptor subtype was discovered and later found to occur throughout the immune system and other peripheral tissues. While scientists were solving old mysteries about cannabis, a new and bigger question was emerging. What physiological purpose do these receptors serve? Nature wouldn't conserve them unless they performed a natural physiological function important to human existence.

As we learn more, it becomes increasingly clear that we are creations of intelligent powers. Our bodies are designed to function with the elements on earth that are provided by God. Attempts to identify endogenous substances that activate these receptors began in the mid-90's and soon culminated in the discovery of numerous other cannabinoids. Since these landmark contributions, ample research has established that the role of the endocannabinoid system is to maintain homeostasis or balance. It ensures that cells communicate effectively, but not excessively.

The Endocannabinoid System (ECS) is a biological system of receptors and neurotransmitters found throughout the brains and nervous systems of all mammalian species. The ECS is the largest biological system of receptors in the body. It holds the potential to revolutionize the ways in which we view health and wellness understanding. The ECS was discovered with scientists studying how cannabis produces effects in the body. Endocrine evidence and receptors bind and exist throughout the body, including the nervous system, immune cells organs, and the brain's connective tissues. The ECS permeates all 11 main physiological systems in the body, working to handle the many functions necessary for survival. The ECS tunes are vital physiological functions. It promotes homeostasis, affecting everything from sleep, appetite, pain, inflammation, memory, mood, and reproduction. The ECS helps to regulate homeostasis across all the major physiological systems, ensuring they're all working in harmony with one another.

The Endocannabinoid System (ECS) comprises three primary components. They are cannabinoids, enzymes, and receptors. Cannabinoids are groups of active compounds that interact with ECS receptors. Indoor cannabinoids are produced naturally inside of the body, while compounds found outside the body, like cannabidiol (CBD) and Tetrahydrocannabinol (THC) are exogenous cannabinoids. CBD is a phytochemical, which means that it originates from plants.

Cannabinoids act as the keys within the endowment cannabinoids system, while receptors act like locks. Every time one key fits into one lock, the lock causes an effect to occur in the body. The main types of endocrines found in the body are for managing appetite, pain response, and immune system functions.

Anandamide commonly referred to as the voice molecule, is responsible for the runner side and the blissful states that come from structured play. Yoga and meditation enzymes or any substance within the body that cause chemical reactions to occur. Enzymes act within the ECS to recycle used cannabinoids after the body is still with them. Receptors receive messages transmitted by cannabinoids. There are two main types of receptors: CB1 and CB2 receptors. CB1 receptors exist in the brain and spinal cord, working to regulate appetite memory and to reduce pain. CB2 receptors are within the immune system and many other areas of the body, working primarily to reduce inflammation throughout the body. Inflammation is a process the body undergoes to heal infected or damaged areas in the body. Inflammation is a main cause of many medical conditions.

In each part of the body, the endocannabinoid system performs different tests, but the ECS always has one goal in mind homeostasis. Your ECS works to keep a stable internal environment through the inevitable changes and variations in the external environment.

It is important to understand that the body produces the cannabinoids necessary to function from normal nutrition. While we understand the impact of THC and CBD, there are up to one hundred or more that we do not yet understand. God made our bodies to function from the nutrition we intake. The use of cannabis could be correctly classified as a nutritional supplement.

As our society and cultures advance, it becomes clearer that we are the result of a mastermind that created us. We are now understanding facts that have been part of our existence for thousands of years.

The discovery of DNA is a perfect example of how our existence is engineered and planned. DNA numbers are much like serial numbers that identify individual items produced with common characteristics.

The future will produce an understanding that will improve humanity more than we ever thought possible. We are all children of God created in his image, but we are still young in his timeline for eternity.

Chapter Three

Addiction and Withdrawal

Addiction is a word that is misunderstood by everyone. The fact is, everyone is addicted to something, whether it be a substance or a habit. The negative thoughts of addiction are associated with substances both dangerous and harmful. For example, heroin is a dangerous drug that can permanently damage you or cause your death. Likewise, addiction to gambling is considered a behavior that must be controlled. When you hear the word addict, these come to mind. Many less dangerous and more normal habits are also actually addictive. The definition of addiction is simply dependency. When someone develops a dependency on a substance or habit, they become addicted to it. Some of the most problematic addictions today are prescribed medications.

Withdrawal, on the other hand, is what happens to our bodies and minds when we stop the use of a substance or the practice of a habit. In the case of highly addictive drugs such as heroin and opioid withdrawal, it is the dangerous part of it that is addiction. One of the most well-known addictions is alcoholism. People behave very irrationally and sometimes offensively when using alcohol. Once they become physically dependent on the substance, withdrawal can be painful. On the other hand, something as simple as sugar can be addictive, but withdrawal is simply resisting a craving.

Another prominent addiction is cigarettes. I personally stopped smoking over 30 years ago. The craving for cigarettes was difficult to resist, and it took me several tries to be successful. The withdrawal from cigarettes was more painful than smoking them, and since cigarette smoking was socially acceptable, it was difficult to want to stop smoking.

Marijuana has been said by some not to be addictive, but I want to assure you once you start using marijuana on a regular basis, you will become addicted. One reason many people say it is not addictive is that withdrawal for an occasional user is not difficult. I will outline the typical withdrawal symptoms of marijuana in this chapter.

One thing that is common to all addictions is that a person must want to stop the addiction to stop. When they stop because a spouse or legal authority requires it, they may not share the desire necessary deep inside. Unless a person is sincerely ready to stop using any addictive substance or habit, they will not endure the withdrawal necessary to accomplish this. It is important to realize that dangerous addictions may require medical assistance to accomplish a safe withdrawal. The root of today's opioid crisis is that it is difficult to stop because doctors prescribe it for pain and those addicted fear the pain will return if they stop. Also, most doctors do not understand that when addicted, it is almost impossible to use in moderation.

Alcoholics Anonymous is a well-known program to help alcoholics stop drinking. They have a 12-step program, which is a spiritual program. It provides spiritual support for those who desire to stop the use of alcohol.

I have personally attended Alcoholics Anonymous meetings to stop my addiction to alcohol. I have also stopped smoking cigarettes after smoking for many years. So why have I not been able to stop smoking marijuana for 50 years? The answer is simple. I have not wanted to stop until now. In all my experience with addiction, both personally and through observation of others, the deep desire to stop is needed to accomplish stopping.

Marijuana is the least addictive and has the less painful withdrawal symptoms of all the mind-altering drugs. It also has many positive advantages that are often preferred over the negative points. I have made the decision now because of several conditions. I will call them long-term side effects that may exist. Research today is not conclusive.

I use the Internet and YouTube for research. Recently, I saw reports of what is called Cannabinoid Hyperemesis Syndrome (CHS). This is a condition where you randomly vomit and cannot control it. Severe cases suffer for days at a time. I have had that condition on several occasions during the last few months. I charged it off to something I ate, but after seeing the YouTube reports, I thought I may have early signs of this condition. I have had other conditions with dry eye, a chronic leg infection, and fatigue that my doctors cannot explain. So, my stopping Cannabis at this time is my own experiment to determine if these conditions will improve.

THC addiction, according to a major study, 70.4% of people struggling with THC addiction will relapse to alleviate THC withdrawal symptoms. Since I have stopped many times throughout my life, I have experienced most of these in the past and returned to its use. The reports about CHS suggest it may take months for the ECS to return to its natural condition. I am prepared to wait for that to happen.

I do attribute other positive conditions to being cured by cannabis. They are arthritis, tooth health, and respiratory health, plus the fact that I have not been required to take many prescription medications, many people my age require. If these conditions return, I may in fact return at some point to cannabis or CBD use in moderation.

The number one withdrawal symptom that people experience when they're going through THC withdrawal is insomnia. Insomnia is particularly annoying because when you are sleep deprived, and you have a lack of sleep, it is proven that your will power also goes down and this makes you much more susceptible to giving in to those cravings, or those moments where you want to relapse.

Symptom number two of THC withdrawal is that you are going to experience excessive sweating. My whole body was just constantly clammy for a few days. This is your body trying to detox the THC that is still circulating in your system.

The third symptom of THC withdrawal is cravings. Cravings are common when you are first quitting THC. Craving is the hardest symptom to resist because it will occur repeatedly, without warning, for some time. Most substance withdrawals will experience cravings. They will make you particularly susceptible to relapse. The only way I have been able to survive those urges is simply to pray to God to get past them. They do eventually stop, but at first, they are just less frequent. About the time you think you have made it; they will grab you and you will relapse.

Symptom number four is irritability and mood changes. For most people, this resembles or comes out in the form of anger. We grow really frustrated quickly, especially with those people who we are closest. Tell people if you are comfortable telling others that you are coming off this substance. You might want to make them aware so they can be prepared and gain a better understanding as to why you are lashing out. The other thing that goes along with irritability and mood changes is that feeling of restlessness or complete loss of concentration and even depression. It will pass, just be ready for it. Again, prayer helps.

Symptom number five is nausea; the endocannabinoid system regulates your digestive system, and that includes feelings of nausea. A lot of people, when they first start quitting cannabis, are unable to eat food. They experience decreased appetite in the first few days and up to the first few weeks due to this intense feeling of nausea.

Symptom number six goes hand in hand with nausea and involves constipation and/or diarrhea.

Symptom number seven that you can anticipate is increased anxiety or increased feelings of depression. This is quite common because, again, your endocannabinoid System (ECS) regulates feelings of anxiety and mood control. Do not be surprised if you are anxious or depressed; these feelings of anxiousness and depression are often heightened by your cravings. You are craving a substance you are not giving your body. That craving you are experiencing is a withdrawal symptom, so of course, in the beginning, you are going to have some feelings of heightened anxiety and even depression.

Symptom number eight is flu-like symptoms. This can include sweating and a slightly increased body temperature. But of course, make sure you do not have COVID-19. Always talk to your doctor when you have a fever. Muscle pain, bone pain and joint pain are included. Just like the flu, you are sick when you are quitting an addiction, whether it is THC, alcohol, or whatever. It may be your body detoxing. You are not going to feel good; it may not be the flu, and I promise this too will pass. If you are detoxing from alcohol as well and are having severe symptoms, especially fever, do not hesitate to contact your doctor or a medically supervised clinic because that can prevent a more serious condition.

Symptom nine is boredom. This is not really a symptom of THC withdrawal, but it is worth mentioning. You are giving up something that was consuming a large part of your day and you are going to find yourself not knowing what to do with your time. Not knowing what to do with this newfound sobriety. When you get bored, you might be inclined to relapse. One thing that will help is to get plenty of rest and, as always, prayer.

Now, the next question naturally becomes, how long is this going to last. Well, most symptoms of THC withdrawal are going to subside somewhere after about four weeks. It has been shown in some studies that it takes much longer for the cannabinoid receptors in your body that THC binds to, to return to their natural levels. For most individuals, peak withdrawals are going to taper off after about four to six weeks. Quitting THC, expect days three to five to be the most challenging. I personally feel that it may take me, as a longtime user, much longer to return to a natural condition. My use has extended over 50 years only with occasional detoxification. The only solid advice I can offer that will help you through this is to stay in prayer and trust God for each step. As I write this chapter, I am in my fifth week of withdrawal. I am doing fine, but I can feel the changes as they occur and sometimes the cravings are almost impossible to resist. I know prayer is what gets me past it.

I know there is a light at the end of the tunnel. Symptoms that people experience include headache, muscle pain, nausea, dizziness, and insomnia are all very physical symptoms, but these usually last only a few weeks. But some people will experience something called pause or post-acute withdrawal symptoms, and these can start once you think they have ended and last anywhere from three months, six months, or longer. You might experience these symptoms on and off for up to a year after quitting using marijuana products. Don't let that scare you. We have seen people quit and still test positive for THC 90 days (about 3 months) after. Especially long-time heavy users and people using concentrates, dabs, and high concentration edible products.

In the years I smoked, I did not feel marijuana could damage me permanently in any way. However, I recognized that when using marijuana; I experienced a false sense of well-being that threatened my ability to be a responsible businessperson. So, I was complacent about periodic use in place of total abstinence. I practiced moderation.

The 12-step program at Alcoholics Anonymous helped me for years after I first went. I managed to control my use of alcohol. I substituted marijuana for the substance I used as a crutch for my emotions. I did learn that to mix the two was a disaster. I must say that the 12-step program led me to accept God as my mediator and, I feel, a relationship with God is essential to overcome any addictive concern.

It is important to understand that God is everywhere and with you all the time. You access him with prayer followed by meditation. His desire for your life is simply to have a relationship with him. It's his desire for you to experience life at its fullest. He wants you to live with the desires in your heart.

I believe God is the creator and mastermind of the universe. All things work together for his glory. The substance that you are addicted to is not the cause of your addiction. It is the excessive use of it that caused your addiction. Moderation in all things is the key to peace within. When you are addicted to something, you must practice total abstinence to restore your natural condition before any consideration is given to moderation. I think the reason the medical profession is having such a crisis with opioids is a lack of understanding of this simple fact. If you must stop the use permanently, God will guide you. I know I cannot smoke cigarettes or drink alcohol again. God has removed my desire.

Chapter Four
Prohibition, Prisons & FDA

In 1936, our government introduced propaganda called "Reefer Madness" to justify the prohibition of Cannabis. In 1937, the Marijuana Tax Act was signed into law by President Roosevelt. Although a study requested by New York City Mayor Fiorello La Guardia found that marijuana wasn't that dangerous, the era of prohibition of cannabis began and continues today on a federal level. Currently, in 2022, legislation is pending in Congress that may finally eliminate it.

In 1951, the United States Congress passed the Boggs Act, which created a mandatory minimum prison sentence for all drug crimes. Five years later, they passed the Narcotics Control Act, which gave stricter mandatory sentences for marijuana-related offenses. Because of this, marijuana became a huge underground activity. Those associated with this counterculture or culture going against mainstream culture consumed it. By the 1950s, marijuana was so taboo, it became a symbol of rebellion against authority. Most importantly, marijuana was regularly lumped into the same category as more dangerous drugs, like heroin and cocaine. The rest of the world fell in line with the stricter marijuana policies of the United States. The 1961 United Nations convention on dark drugs created a rule that marijuana should be banned unless it was used for strictly medical purposes or scientific research. Every country now was on board in the late 1960s. The American counterculture movement associated with hippies and college students grew dramatically, and they liked marijuana. Meanwhile, soldiers were taking marijuana and all kinds of drugs during the Vietnam War. This freaked many Americans out. In 1968, Richard Nixon, who promised to restore law and order, was elected president, partially due to this freaking out by the people. In 1969, the Supreme Court found that the Marijuana Tax Act was unconstitutional because it violated the 5th Amendment. In response, Congress passed the Controlled Substances Act. This placed drugs into categories based on how dangerous they were. Drugs classified as Schedule One are the most dangerous. The law placed marijuana as a Schedule One drug and therefore eligible for the heaviest restrictions and penalties. Now marijuana was officially banned and completely illegal in all cases in the United States. The next year, the United Kingdom followed suit, but classified marijuana as less dangerous than other drugs. Back in the United States, a group called NORML, which stands for the National Organization for the

Reform of Marijuana Laws, was established to end marijuana prohibition. Their support and influence quickly grew. In 1972, the Shafer Commission created by President Nixon found that marijuana wasn't as dangerous as other Schedule One drugs, and suggested marijuana be decriminalized or have the penalties less harsh. Nixon ignored their suggestion. The Nixon administration, as it turns out, found it convenient to keep marijuana illegal to control those darn hippies. In fact, Nixon declared a full-on war on drugs; he created the DEA or Drug Enforcement Administration. In 1975, the Supreme Court ruled 20 years in prison for having marijuana was okay, even though many states wanted to decriminalize marijuana. Marijuana use continued to increase during the rest of the decade. In 1976, the Netherlands decriminalized marijuana. For the longest time, it was the only place in the entire world where you could consume marijuana and not get in big trouble. Then another backlash, a grassroots movement, began against marijuana. Conservative parent organizations were lobbying the government for stricter regulation and more propaganda to prevent teenagers from using it. By the time Ronald Reagan was elected president in 1980, the culture was changing again. This time turning against marijuana, yet again, during the 1980s, anti-drug propaganda was at its height, from the just-say-no campaign to DARE. The partnership for a drug free America. Nobody, like your lawyer or your local police officer, would say marijuana was harmless. The Reagan administration started locking up more people for using it and making the punishments even more severe. This propaganda did not differentiate marijuana from more dangerous drugs, and marijuana continued to be attacked and feared by most. In the 1980s and 1990s, law enforcement across the United States cracked down hard on marijuana users. Minorities were disproportionately targeted even though they did not use it any more than non-minorities. Millions still call for making medical marijuana legal. In 1996, California passed proposition 250, which legalized medical marijuana. Once again, there were several other states that soon followed. By the late 1990s, anti-marijuana propaganda had faded, and more films featured regular marijuana use. Again, more studies and doctors began to call for decriminalization and for legal medical use. Many countries around the world did just that. Portugal famously not only decriminalized marijuana, but decriminalized all drugs and crime associated with drugs. In 2001, Canada legalized medical marijuana across the country. American politicians ignored them despite a new War on Terror after the horrific 9/11 attacks. Hundreds of thousands of marijuana dealers and sellers in the United States were arrested each year in the

2000s. Shortly after, President Barack Obama took office in 2009. Obama once wrote about how he used to smoke marijuana when he was a teenager. By this time in the Obama administration, more people were now calling for recreational marijuana to be legalized. Several countries had legalized medical marijuana even though the European Union (EU) government had remained strict about enforcing marijuana laws. On November 6th, 2012, both Colorado and Washington said we do not care and completely legalized marijuana for adults after seeing how much money they could make from taxing it and regulating it. Realizing the effects of legalization were not as bad as previously thought; a wave of others also sought to legalize it recreationally. In 2013, Uruguay became the first country to legalize marijuana for adults 18 years and older. Cannabis was legal in every country in the world until the 20th century, and I predict, that within a decade, it will be legal in every country in the world again. The changing worldwide culture has dramatically shifted as people have learned the facts about marijuana. Now that we have seen the success of marijuana legalization, there really is no going back. That said, moderation is the key to preventing addiction. I feel it is the excessive use of anything that causes problems.

Prohibition of marijuana started with misinformation as an effort to stop the industrial development of industrial cannabis. Giant leaders and politicians led the movement to protect their own interests, which were invested in alternative methods. The misinformation may have continued to protect those who were invested in private prison systems. The United States has 5% of the world's population and 23% of the world's prison population. Could it be that our politicians and their influencers are profiting from these private prisons? A sizable portion of our prison population is the result of drug enforcement.

Big Pharma profits from manufacturing drugs that can be patented and sold at a premium price. A plant that may even be grown by an individual does not offer any potential profit to Big Pharma. Could payoffs and lobbyists to politicians be a factor in why cannabis has been banned so long?

The FDA started in 1906 to protect people against harmful foods and drugs. This was originally prompted by the considerable number of products being sold without any restriction and some being harmful or misrepresented as to the benefits.

Society has advanced and grown, and the role of the FDA has changed into a bureaucracy that employs about 18,000 people (about the seating capacity of Madison Square Garden) today. Some substances that are regulated by the FDA today do not require approval. An example of non-approved items that the FDA regulates are sold as food supplements and vitamins. These items must be labeled accurately as to the contents and make no claim as to any benefits.

Drugs and some devices intended for medical use are not only regulated but must also be approved before they can be sold. These must undergo testing before they are approved and contain labels and warnings that tell any side effects discovered by testing.

The FDA does not actually do the testing. They approve drugs based on tests provided by the seller or advocate of the substance. The seller's test will include recommended labeling and dosage recommendations for the desired result. The only role the FDA plays is to provide approval.

In 1970, the government classified marijuana as a Schedule One drug, along with heroin and LSD. This classification designates the substance as dangerous, with a high likelihood of abuse and no apparent medical advantage. These drugs warrant the most severe penalties under the law. This is often given as a reason that more research has not been accomplished on cannabis.

However, one of the most serious drug problems in society today is the opioid crisis. Opioids are from the same plant as heroin, also a Schedule One drug. So, the question becomes how research on a Schedule One drug heroin results in FDA approval when cannabis has not.

I cannot offer direct proof, and my opinion can only be speculative as a reason. The original motivation for the prohibition of cannabis was partially because drug makers wanted it banned because manufactured drugs in a laboratory were more profitable. Many of the drugs available today not only originate in the laboratory but are patented, which makes them even more expensive. The FDA requires extensive testing, which is also costly. The only people who can justify that cost are the large pharmaceutical companies who can realize large profits from patented drugs. These companies also have deep pockets and can lobby politicians for favorable legislation.

I feel the real cancer today in society is corruption. A large bureaucracy is a breeding ground for corruption. The annual profits from opioids for Big Pharma today are estimated to exceed $35 billion (about $110 per person in the US). Another interesting statistic is that states that have legalized marijuana for medical purposes have seen a reduction in opioid overdoses of 23%. Cannabis can be used to relieve pain instead of an opioid. My experience of using cannabis for arthritis pain eventually cured the arthritis. I do not think a pain killer will do that. The profits from cannabis sales, a plant, do not offer the same potential profit as those from manufactured drugs. This is a simple reason we have not tested cannabis.

Chapter Five
Industrial Hemp & Reefer Madness

So absurd and untenable has become the government's position on marijuana that more people are beginning to suspect that Reefer Madness, the prohibition of cannabis, is not based on the presumed dangers of its chemical compounds but on the tremendous potential that hemp has always shown in history for industrial production. In ancient times as the miracle plant, the sister of man, a gift from the gods, the history of cannabis has been deeply linked to human history since the dawn of civilization. The cannabis plant has been an invaluable source to produce textiles, paper, food, and fuel, in addition to providing a wide range of important medicinal remedies. The cannabis plant is very resistant, can grow at almost any latitude, requires no pesticides to be cultivated, and grows faster than all other crops. Cannabis can produce up to 25 tons of biomass a year per cultivated acre. The two most common species of cannabis are sativa and indica. The first one taller and slender, has thinner foliage and can reach up to 24 feet in height. Indica is much stockier and thicker and foliage also thus sativa leaves are thinner and more elongated, while those of the indica are shorter and more well-rounded. A third type of cannabis less common is ruderalis, which grows in the colder regions of Central Asia. The chemical compound causing the mental alterations in the smoker called THC is found only in the leaf and flower of cannabis. The rest of the plant can be used to derive hundreds of useful products without having to discard a single gram of the stock. Cannabis is composed of an inner, woodier, rigid part, and an outer wrapping, which is softer and fibrous in nature. The central stem of the pulp for paper production. The oldest cannabis paper dates to the Chinese empire of 6000 B.C. In Europe, the use of cannabis paper began in the 8th century under the emperor Charlemagne, who strongly encouraged its cultivation. It was used by monks to copy the holy scriptures. Cannabis paper also provided the parchments for the first Bible printed by Gutenberg. The outer wrapping of the stem produces the fiber needed to make ropes and fabrics which are universally recognized for their quality and durability. Millions of miles of rope of all types and sizes have been produced with cannabis fiber in the course of history. The range of fabrics that can be produced with a fiber of cannabis is virtually unlimited. The beauty of hemp fiber is that it can be many things depending on its method of cultivation and the method of processing. These can range from course hessians, industrial fabrics, such as carpet backings, to the finest linens. Cannabis fabrics are softer and stronger than cotton. They cost less, and their manufacturing, unlike cotton, produces no pollution. The seeds of cannabis can be used as a food base. They can be ground into a high protein flour or used to produce an excellent edible oil rich in protein carbohydrates and essential fatty acids, such as Omega 3 and Omega 6. The oil of cannabis may also provide a superior fuel for illumination and domestic heating, or it can be used as fuel for cars in the form of ethanol. There is no smoke emitting from this oil, as it is clean burning.

It is an excellent fuel for cars. The manufacturer, Henry Ford, decided to build a prototype automobile that was built entirely with vegetable products, especially cannabis and its derivatives. The engine was already using a blend of 10% ethanol, while the body was made up of a special biodegradable plastic much lighter but significantly stronger than a normal metallic body.

In fact, there are at least 5000 items that could be produced with cannabis. Among these are crackers, animal cages, insulation materials, textile fibers, guitar cases, sheets, rollers, mascara, napkins, oatmeal, mattresses, footwear, T-shirts, shoelaces, earmuffs, diapers, baby pacifiers, pillows, hammocks, speaker boxes, shower curtains, chairs, deodorants, blankets, drums, coffee filters, clogs, sawdust for the stalls, curtains, hats, boots, ironing boards, underwear, towels, clubs, candles, surfboards, and even houses can be built in large part with cannabis products.

Despite this, the production of cannabis is currently banned everywhere in the world. The problems with cannabis began in the 1930s in the wake of the industrial revolution.

A new movement in America was born that listed Henry Ford among its founders. Instead of abandoning agriculture to itself and directing all investments toward industry, this movement sought to transform and to harness agricultural output to integrate it into industrial production. The idea was to use agricultural products, cannabis, to provide the industry with all the raw materials it needed. But there was a major handicap in making the production of cannabis truly competitive. The separation of the fiber from the stock still needed to be done by hand, and this slowed down production, increasing the cost.

But the invention of a new machine the decorticator hemp machine. It removed the last barrier for cannabis. Finally, promising unlimited success at that time. The magazine Popular Mechanics published a landmark article entitled "New Billion Dollar Crop" in which it had a vision of a tremendous revival of cannabis plantations all around the world.

Not everyone was happy with the future success of this miracle plant at that time. The magnet of pink journalism, William Randolph Hearst, had bought millions of acres of timber forests which he intended to use to make paper for his ever more popular tabloid publications. With the return of hemp paper, far less expensive than tree paper, his empire was doomed to collapse in a fleeting period. Another industry giant who was directly threatened by the return of cannabis was Lamont DuPont. He was the owner of a petrochemical company that had just bought the patents to create dozens of synthetic products from oil. He was to make nylon stockings, brushes, men's clothing, tires, Orlon, Dacron, synthetic sponges, cellophane, and a full range of products that would have been easily displaced on the market by their competitors made with hemp. Apart from the risk of losing millions of dollars, Hearst and DuPont had something else in common. They were both funded by one of the most powerful bankers of the time, Andrew Mellon. Andrew Mellon was also the owner of Gulf Oil, one of the so-called Seven Sisters. At that time, oil companies were expanding at great speed, but were likely to see their investments vanish by the mass production of cannabis, which offered a much cleaner and more economical fuel.

We should not forget the young pharmaceutical industry, which was financed by two other powerful bankers, John Rockefeller, and Andrew Carnegie. These people were conducting an all-out campaign to eliminate accepted natural herbal treatments, including cannabis from the pharmacopeia, while trying to replace them with drugs created in the laboratory. Furthermore, Rockefeller was also the owner of Standard Oil, which had already started to invade America with its refineries and its service stations.

Thus, was born in this natural alliance between the paper, synthetic textile, the oil industry, the producers of plastics and its derivatives, and the pharmaceutical industry. They all needed to get rid of the common enemy as soon as possible. Luckily for them, at that time, Andrew Mellon was also the secretary of the treasury. From that powerful position, he appointed his future son-in-law, Terry Anslinger, to be the Head of The New Federal Bureau of Narcotics. Harry Anslinger had already had experience as a federal agent during prohibition. His job was now to transform the crumbling bureaucracy of alcohol prohibition, which had been abolished, into a new weapon to combat and eradicate cannabis from a future in this nation. He said, "My department intends to pursue a relentless warfare against the despicable dope peddling boxer who preys on the weakness of his fellow man. "

However, he could not open the attack on cannabis, which was a plant loved and respected by the vast majority. Anslinger had the brilliant idea of using the Mexican nickname marijuana. This was unknown to Americans at the time. In doing so, on the one hand, he managed to divert suspicions of the true objectives of the operation. On the other, by attaching the use of marijuana to Black people and Mexicans, it made it much easier to ride the growing wave of racism that was already sweeping across the country. Adding coal to the fire, Anslinger declared that marijuana is mostly used by Black people, Hispanics, Filipinos, and entertainers. Their satanic music, jazz, and swing results from marijuana use. This marijuana causes white women to seek sexual relations with the negroes, entertainers, and many others. The backlash was immediate and soon a new green monster was born. The market was flooded with publications of all kinds in which marijuana also known as reefer. It became synonymous with sin, moral depravity, violence, recklessness, and even murder. From the most popular tabloids to adventure books; from comic strips to sophisticated magazines such as, Cosmopolitan. All owned by Randolph Hearst. There was hardly a publication that did not join the cause of demonizing marijuana.

Now that puritan America had found its enemy, Anslinger felt it was time to extend the fear to the entire population. America was threatened by a new drug menace. Street corner vendors would stock in trade the deadly local weed, marijuana. Pass it out in cigarette form from ingeniously concealed containers. The referrers go to the waiting hands of diluted youngsters. The dried leaves and flowers of the Hemp Dogbane, also known as, Indian hemp weed, were used in the form of a cigarette. Marijuana smoking, experts point out, can make a helpless addict a victim within weeks, causing physical and moral ruin, and even death. Every week, he loaded them with false reality and fear of brutality, murders, sex crimes, insanity, or suicide, should you ever be confronted with the temptation of taking that first puff of a marijuana cigarette.

At the end of this devastatingly effective media campaign, a bill was introduced in Congress that in fact prohibited the cultivation and use of marijuana, even though its psychotropic compounds are found only in the flowers and leaves. Cannabis was to have the entire cultivation of the plant prohibited. Across the country, most of the representatives and senators who voted on the bill, in fact, did not even know that cannabis and marijuana were the same thing. At that time, congress people voting on legislation were not aware that marijuana was hemp cannabis. Hemp that the country had been using profitably for centuries without public debate.

Without the support of scientific research, in 1937, the Marijuana Tax Act was approved by President Roosevelt. The war on cannabis had officially begun. There were dozens of glamorous arrests which the same Hurst immediately made known to the entire nation.

Not everyone believed in the demonic dangers of marijuana. The popular mayor of New York City, Fiorello LaGuardia, commissioned a scientific investigation to ascertain the real effects of marijuana on the user. Thirty-one independent scientists worked for over five years, completing what became the first known scientific study on the use of marijuana. It was published in 1944. The LaGuardia report showed surprising results. Marijuana, it said, does not cause aggressive or antisocial behavior. Does not cause an increase in sexual depravity. Does not alter the fundamental aspects of personality.

Furious, Anslinger immediately resorted to the press to discredit the research. Then unleashed his agents all over the country with the task of destroying every copy of the report they could find. Still not satisfied, Anslinger steered the media propaganda so that casual smokers of marijuana became associated with users of hard drugs such as heroin, cocaine, or morphine. It is a symbol, a symbol of narcotic addictions poisoning the blood of our country. When the addict is deprived of their addiction, they experience withdrawal symptoms. They live from fix to fix. The addict must have their drug, and to get it, they must have money, and that much money comes hard. Marijuana is the most prevalent narcotic among juveniles. Its greatest danger lies in the fact that it is a steppingstone to hard drugs such as morphine and heroin. 95% of narcotic addicts begin with the use of marijuana based on this myth, which has never been confirmed by scientific research. The marijuana user was associated with the figure of the pathetic drug addict. The social reject, the loser who no longer had a chance of recovery.

Building on this misinformation campaign, as Anslinger convinced Congress to enact a new life, which provided that the smoker of marijuana would suffer the same penalties as that of hard drug users such as cocaine or heroin. In 1956, the first arrest for possession of marijuana carried a mandatory sentence of two to ten years in prison. In some states, like Missouri, a second arrest for marijuana possession could be punished with life behind bars.

Now that America was under control, Anslinger turned his attention to the rest of the world. Cannabis was still being cultivated freely around the world. At the United Nations, Anslinger began knitting a Machiavellian web of diplomacy. The United States could now exert influence over other nations. In 1961, Anslinger culminated his career by persuading the UN to unify all single existing treaties on drug control. Thus, was born, the single convention for narcotic drugs to which more than 150 countries adhered. They established an international tribunal with the control of drugs and committed individual states, among other things, to combat and eradicate as soon as possible the cultivation of cannabis. Within a few years, the production of cannabis would become illegal virtually everywhere in the world.

The petrochemical industry had won its battle. While the world received in exchange, the huge ecological disaster we are witnessing today. Air pollution, the contamination of aquifers, rivers, and the seabed. Wild deforestation, extinction of animal species, global warming, and most importantly, our slavery to oil, which could be erased at any time by simply going back to cannabis as the basis for all fuel production.

One hundred years ago, the farmer produced all the fiber, all the medicine, all the fuel, and all the food that was consumed. That is what our economy is. You raise those four basic categories, fiber, food, medicine, and fuel, and you sell them to the necessities of life. To me, that sounds like God's plan. The money flows out from the city to the landowners and those responsible for production of wealth. It has been that way for thousands of years.

Today, 100 years later, the farmer does not produce any fiber. If they do, it is with cotton, which accounts for 50% of the pesticides and herbicides used in the agricultural sector. The farmer does not raise any medicine. It has all been monopolized by pharmaceutical companies who manufacture medicines in a laboratory. The farmer does not raise fuel. It's all extracted from natural resources by petrol and chemical companies. Go into the grocery store and look at the ingredients on the package. You will find out how radically farmers are being displaced from the heritage of food production. It has all been taken over by processed food, the synthetic manufacturers who, in producing these products, create the toxic waste.

Today, much of the focus is still on the debate about the recreational use of cannabis and its value in medicines. The real story of cannabis is still being hidden. The potential to restore an eco-friendly source for many of our modern needs is to restore industrial use of cannabis. The movement of electric vehicles and solar power is not really an eco-friendly solution to our concerns about climate change. In fact, raw materials for batteries are not plentiful in the United States. The real movement to electric vehicles may be more an effort to shift economic strength to China than a concern about the environment.

Cannabis, on the other hand, can be produced in every country and could serve as an economic balance for our world. With legalization, the missing link remains the infrastructure necessary to process farm production. It may take years before we see a practical use of industrial hemp again for many products. Other countries are also being led by leaders with corrupt self-interest as well. Hemp has the potential to fix many problems people face. Hopefully, corrupt lawmakers will not prevail.

One of the first products to be processed from industrial hemp today is CBD. Industrial hemp is both low in THC content and high in CBD content. It is an excellent source for CBD and is now legal to grow in the United States.

The Magic & Mystery of Marijuana

Chapter Six
CBD Products

The legalization of marijuana has set a legal guideline based on THC content of the cannabis plant. The cannabis plant has around forty different strains worldwide, all with different properties. To understand the differences, think of citrus fruits. All are similar, but each individual strain is uniquely different. THC and CBD have become known as a substance used in the newly discovered endocannabinoid system. This is an important system in our bodies that wasn't known before 1964 and was not really researched much until the mid-1990s. This system in our bodies uses about one hundred different cannabinoids to accomplish critical functions in our bodies known as homeostasis. This means cellular balance. It affects every cell in our bodies. THC is the only cannabinoids that affect us in a psychotropic way, which means it gets us high. The other cannabinoids serve other purposes and do not get you high. CBD has been determined to have many benefits to our bodies without the psychotropic properties, so it is legal to sell or consume when the THC is not present. Some strains of cannabis contain exceptionally low levels of THC and higher levels of CBD. While CBD can be extracted from most strains, the content of THC associated with it can make some extractions illegal to sell. It is possible to extract only the CBD from a plant, and that is known as an isolate, which is pure CBD.

Other extraction methods will extract all the properties in a plant along with the CBD and are known as full spectrum. The full spectrum contains an array of other cannabinoids and terrines not yet understood. When the plant contains a low level of THC, naturally, it can be sold legally as CBD. These extractions are from industrial hemp. There is much controversy about what is best to use and not everyone agrees about any option. Not only will pure CBD isolate not get you high, but it will also not test positive in a drug test. Full Spectrum, on the other hand, contains not only CBD, but all the properties of a plant. While it may not contain enough THC to get you high or be illegal, it may trigger a drug test as positive.

Since strains vary and growing conditions cause differences in plants, not all full spectrum extractions will be the same. When using CBD full spectrum, you may experience different results from different batches. The government requires the absence of pesticides and an accurate description as to CBD and THC content, but evaluation as to the content of other cannabinoids contained is not present. Most users agree the full spectrum provides more benefits. The cannabinoids work together in an entourage effect to produce results.

My use of marijuana for many years was strictly for recreational use. When I was in my fifties, I developed arthritis with knee pain at first. My doctor prescribed Celebrex for it and it eased the pain. When Celebrex was banned for use by the FDA, I was prescribed other pain medications that never seemed to help as much. By the time I reached sixty years old, I realized marijuana was a better pain reliever than the pain medications I was prescribed, so I rarely used them, and was content with marijuana.

When I learned about CBD, I was anxious to try it. At that time, a small bottle was about $100, and the instructions were to use a few drops under your tongue at bedtime. By this time, my arthritis not only was in my knees, but my hands, and elbows. My knuckles were swollen, and nodes were apparent to them. Within a few days, I noticed greater pain relief than ever experienced with pain medications or just marijuana. I then obtained CBD from several sources and did some research. The pain relief alone was enough to get me interested, but some claims were that CBD would address the problem in addition to relief of the pain. I have used it long enough to know that is true. There was no clear information about dosage except to say you couldn't overdose on it. I shopped around and became a dealer to resell a product known as Holy Grail. It was manufactured by a small California company that obtained its raw product from a small grower in Colorado. While I did sell these products, my main objective was to get my own costs lower. I began using about 250mg (about the weight of ten grains of rice) daily. The immediate results were noticeable, and the added benefit was noticed with my teeth. I had been experiencing tooth pain with gums that had receded and thought I would lose my teeth soon. I continued this dosage for a few years.

I had an injury when I was thirteen years old when I was hit by a car. I spent most of ninth grade in the hospital and had massive tissue loss and a broken leg. I fully recovered from this but have a large scar on my left leg. I have little feeling about it today. A small growth emerged in the middle of that scar. Doctors would just look at it and tell me we needed to watch it. This went on for over two years. Then one day it erupted, much like a pimple bursting, and it became a large infected sore. X-rays revealed it came from an area near the original break in my leg bone. I was referred to an infectious disease specialist. The original concern was that it might be present in my bones. The good news was it was not. He treated it for about 90 days (about 3 months) with six different antibiotics. While these seemed to help, they in no way cured the problem. The specialist finally told me that he had not been able to find a cause for this; the cultures would not grow, and he did not want to keep me on antibiotics. We discussed the possibility of CBD contributing to this and he said little was known about CBD, but it was possible. He told me he wouldn't tell me to stop the CBD. That was three years ago.

Soon I realized I was feeling very tired and lacked energy. One of the Benefits of CBD is it calms you down. I felt the high dosage of CBD might be the cause of my fatigue. So, I reduced my CBD intake to just 25mg (about the weight of a grain of rice) daily. My leg has continued to improve but still has a small amount of drainage today. In the past, I had a doctor prescribe antibiotics at times for temporary relief. The healing is like waves. It gets almost healed, then it gets worse. Since my nerves in my leg are almost nonexistent, I have little pain with this. As I write this, I am in my seventh week of no CBD or marijuana. My leg has not gotten worse and appears to be improving at the same rate as always.

A miracle today that I attribute to CBD and cannabis is that my arthritis is gone. The swollen knuckles have gone away, and I do not have that pain any longer. Recently, a blood test I had included a test for arthritis. It tested negative, meaning I do not have arthritis any longer. The only question in my mind is would it be gone if I had not taken the high dosage and is it going to return if I stop completely.

Another miracle from CBD use is my teeth. With receded gums, my teeth were exposed below the gum line and damaged from brushing. They are loose and, of course, painful. Today my teeth are solid, and the groves from the damage are gone. I still have my original teeth at age 78.

Now the conditions I feel may have side effects. I have experienced dry eye. Initially, an eye doctor told me I was allergic to smoke. Since I worked in bars as a karaoke host, I was reacting to cigarette smoke. The venue I first experienced it was a smoking bar. I eventually stopped working at that first venue, but the condition continued. I was taking drops that were supposed to help with an allergic reaction.

When I was younger, I had allergies and took shots that cured me. I asked to be tested for allergies. It came back as I had no allergies, so the cause of my dry eye was not allergies. My doctor then tested for other known causes of dry eye and could find no cause. The condition continued to get worse, so I stopped working as a karaoke host in bars and restaurants after eighteen years. Since that time, the condition has not caused a problem. However, stopping my job also changed another habit. I have never smoked marijuana while working or in public.

My habit was to smoke prior to my show and by the time I finished, it had worn off. So, when I got home, I would smoke to unwind before I went to bed. The reaction to dry eye always occurred after I went to bed, or shortly before.

I recently saw a YouTube video that described a condition known as Cannabinoid Hyperemesis Syndrome. This is explained as an uncontrolled urge to vomit that continues uncontrollably. In some cases, this condition is severe. The explanation was that the endocannabinoid system was causing this from too much cannabis intake and the only cure was to stop using cannabis. This video also mentioned that there was a high concentration of these CB receptors in the eye and that red eyes were also associated with this condition.

My experience in marketing CBD was enlightening. Legalization of marijuana and industrial hemp caused something that might be compared to the gold rush. Many companies were formed to take advantage of this new market. Promoters sold stock in these companies, and numerous penny stocks were in existence. A penny stock can exist when a business has a stock valuation that far exceeds the real financial needs of the company. The promoters use the proceeds from stock sales for personal lifestyle and promotion instead of the legitimate needs of the business. When industrial hemp was deemed legal nationwide, these companies saw this as an expanded market and quickly addressed it. The initial introduction of CBD into the market was extremely high in price and very profitable to the promoters. A market was established quickly with prices that were a dollar per ml or higher. This was possible because production was limited, and the product worked miraculously.

As legalization progressed, supply increased rapidly, and price dropped drastically. The market started selling larger quantities at the price points previously used for smaller quantities. In fact, most manufacturers have eliminated the 100ml bottle. The promotion of a higher dosage is not healthy. Legalization without understanding is dangerous. I hope this will be corrected before the benefits are lost from misinformation.

Since doctors do not really want to discuss cannabis- related theories, I must make my choices on my own. There are many positive effects from the use of cannabis, but as with almost any other drug, side effects may occur that are not positive. That is why dosage is so important, and moderation may be good, while in excess, not so good. It is not possible to go from excess to moderation; the excess has already changed your body in response to the substance. I learned that from other addictions.

I have stopped the use of cannabis to enable my body to restore itself to a natural condition. After I have completely removed the toxins etc. from my body, it will be necessary to allow time to restore my natural metabolism. If I use cannabis in the future, it will be in moderation.

Chapter Seven
Restoration Of Our Bodies

God made our bodies to function with the intake of the many nutrients provided here on earth. Our bodies are flexible and can adjust to different combinations of input. Diet is the most important aspect of being healthy. Often misunderstood, our medical system does not treat the root causes of disease, but rather the symptoms. When our body is operating efficiently, the needed nutrients are available from the food we consume, and our immune system and other body systems do the work together to provide a healthy life experience.

With addiction, you are adding a substance that may cause your body to get its metabolism out of balance. Withdrawal is the first reaction when you stop using the addictive substance. As the toxins are removed, a reaction occurs.

After they are removed, the withdrawal symptoms will disappear, but your body may have been damaged by the excesses. The human body is a miracle itself, as it heals itself when given conditions that allow this.

In simple terms, a healthy diet is essential for complete restoration of body functions. With cannabis and the endocannabinoid system, every cell in your body may be impacted. It may take several months before you can experience total recovery and restoration of your body. This will only happen with a healthy diet.

Personally, I have been a student of complete nutrition for years. I have taken a variety of supplements over the years. Before the pandemic, I drank fresh wheatgrass juice daily. I lost my source for this, so today, I drink at least one Ensure shake daily and take some vitamins, minerals, and other supplements. I cannot recommend any specific diet from my experience; in fact, I think constantly trying different supplements is a good practice since there are some that are better than others. However, I am overweight from my ideal weight. I think that may be common with marijuana users, as its use sure makes food taste good. I am going to try a thirty-day Keto diet to lose some weight. Hopefully, I can get back to normal weight soon. I need to lose about fifty pounds to be at my ideal weight.

Our bodies are biological, but as humans, we also have a spirit within us. That is the part of us that is created in God's image. I know we have a direct line to God through prayer. Prayer should be followed by meditation. It is necessary to build on that connection to enjoy life at its fullest. Addiction may be a tool God uses to bring us to that reality. As I age, I find it easier to open my heart to God. The sooner you can do this, the sooner you will find total peace in your life. While churches, twelve-step programs, etc. are good, it is not necessary to participate in any program to open your heart to God. You are a child of God. Jesus is the son of God. His example is total trust in God for the direction of his life. In the next chapter, I will tell my story as it relates to my journey. Cannabis played a vital role for me. I can also see how God has been there for me.

Chapter Eight

My Story

I was born in 1943, but I will start my story with my parents before I was born. They met while attending Texas Tech in Lubbock, Texas. Both had survived the Great Depression. At the time, Lubbock was the home of a new college known as Texas Tech. They moved there to complete their education.

My mom was raised on a farm and had three brothers. Two of her brothers were much younger, and when their mother died of cancer, my mom, being the older girl in the family, became like a mother to her younger brothers. Her dad and her mother both had a lot of brothers, so there were a lot of aunts and uncles and cousins in her family. As for depression, she said they suffered truly little and couldn't tell much difference in life because they lived on a farm. Her stories were about her growing up on a farm.

In those days, a person could get a teaching certificate when they finished high school, and that is what my mom did. She taught school for a family on a ranch before moving to Lubbock to attend Texas Tech. She went to Texas Tech to finish her education and became a teacher at a Lubbock High School. That was in the thirties.

My dad, on the other hand, suffered greatly during the depression. He was from Sherman, Texas, and his dad was a carpenter. My dad also had one older sister. Their mother died from lack of nourishment because of depression. My dad was a young boy without a mother and raised himself. The depression brought challenging times for their family to the point that they were hungry. I really do not know much about his childhood. All I know is that he became an Eagle Scout and spent much of his time in the library reading. He had knowledge of many subjects. His dad was a carpenter and had a problem finding work during the depression.

Eventually, my dad hopped a freight train to get to Lubbock from Sherman so he could go to Texas Tech. When he arrived in Lubbock, he had no money. I know he got assistance from the Salvation Army and eventually he found a boarding house that allowed him to work for his room and board. He attended classes without getting credit because he couldn't afford the tuition. He did this so that he could learn his chosen profession, architecture.

He found work as a draftsman at a local architecture firm who had military contracts during the war. When he could afford to pay the tuition, he would retake a course to get credit for it for graduation. It took him thirteen years to get his degree. He worked his entire life at an architecture firm. He became a partner when he finished his education.

My mom and my dad were married around 1935, and she worked while my dad finished his education. When I was born, they had been married for about seven years. My dad was already well established as an architect, and with the help of his dad, a carpenter, they had already built the house; I grew up in.

When I was born, my mom quit working and was a stay-at-home mom. When I was young, our house was on the edge of town, and I remember the cotton fields behind our house. My earliest memories start when my sister was born. I remember them bringing her home from the hospital and a house cleaner we had that looked like Aunt Jemima was there to help with household duties. I know now that my mom and dad had worked hard to build a home and establish a family that did not have to suffer the way they did during the depression. We were living the American dream.

I will not detail many of the memories of my life here. This is not intended to be my life story, but an understanding of how I managed temptation and addiction with God's help. I will hit the highlights and turning points. My childhood, up until the time

I was a teenager, was a model of the American dream. I was provided with all the innovative technology, from electric trains, tape recorders, model airplanes, electronic gadgets, and photographic equipment, to pets, tropical fish and stamp collecting. I was able to learn about the world of my parents' dreams. I was interested in many things and shared a lot of time with my dad as my teacher until I was about thirteen. I had all the normal childhood diseases and suffered from asthma and allergies.

My mom took care of domestic issues, including sick kids. She was a role model as a stay-at-home mom. Our family had domestic help, and she managed the household to perfection. I never went without anything I needed, and everything had a place. My mom was organized. She was also the spiritual leader in our household. My dad never attended church with us, and I never really understood the reason. When I was around nine years old, I accepted Christ as my savior and was baptized in a Baptist Church. I remember the deep feeling I had at the time. I pretended to be a preacher with an orange crate as my podium and read the Bible to neighborhood children.

Soon, however, I focused my attention on worldly things. I was especially interested in photography and by the time I was ten, had a photographic darkroom in the basement of our house and developed my own pictures. On Saturdays, my dad would take me to a local camera store in downtown Lubbock. I would obtain supplies and more sophisticated equipment on those visits.

The people who owned the camera store had no children of their own and took a special interest in me. I got my first real job with them when I was about 11. I would work on Saturdays at the store. My duties included cleaning and stocking merchandise. These people had a strong influence on me from that time until I was grown.

On the surface, they were kind and responsible people. They communicated that image to my dad. However, there was a dark side to them that led to much confusion in my teenage years. They were alcoholics with some perversion and tempted me in ways that I will not detail except to say they exposed me to the use of alcohol and cigarettes when I was about 12 years old. At that time, I was a technician in their custom photo darkroom and the owner would work in the darkroom with me and make it possible for me to drink alcohol. I also started smoking cigarettes in the darkroom as well. I resisted many temptations that never should be exposed to a young person and kept many incidents a secret.

As I got older, I earned enough money to buy a motor scooter and learned to drive at the early age of 13. On the first day of school, in the ninth grade,

I had an accident on the scooter when a car hit me. This broke my leg and caused a huge tissue loss on my left leg. I spent several months in the hospital before I was able to attend classes at school.

When I returned to school, I met a boy who became one of my best friends. He was also on crutches. He had broken his leg in an accident when he was drunk in a park with some other boys. Lubbock was a dry county and liquor was not sold retail anywhere closer than about 90 miles from Lubbock. Bootleggers were plentiful in Lubbock, and I was introduced to them by my new friend. Soon my weekends were spent hanging out with a group of boys who would go to the bootleggers, and we got drunk. Soon after, three of us became interested in rock-and-roll music and our weekends included playing in bands around the Lubbock area and, of course, alcohol.

I continued to work at the camera store. In high school, I took distributive education, which allowed me to attend school half a day and work in the afternoons at the store for school credit. The dark side of those people at the camera store were adults that encouraged my behavior of drinking and playing rock-and-roll music. Eventually, I was out of control in the eyes of my parents, and with the influence of the camera store owner; I was sent to military school. I feel much of the influence of that camera store owner was fear that his behavior toward me would be revealed if I did not leave town.

Military school was a positive experience. However, many of the cadets were there, as they had also been sent there because they were out of control.

I was not in the official band company, but on one occasion, I sat in with a stage band that was an extension of the band company. This band played country music. I was invited to join the stage band, and because the counselors at Allen Academy were from Texas A&M University; we were allowed to play at some fraternity functions of the college. I was still able to enjoy playing music, but it was more structured, and the music was different. We did manage to find alcohol on some of those events, and I only got caught once. I was given a warning and never suffered any consequences.

Lubbock was a little too far from this school to go home on weekend leaves, so on several occasions I was allowed to go to Houston with some of my friends that lived there. We would party and consume alcohol during those times. In those years, marijuana was not part of the equation, and I was afraid of any drugs.

Military school was a positive experience for me. I managed to get my grades up and graduated from high school as a member of the National Honor Society. I was number thirteen in a graduating class of approximately 100 students. More importantly, I was able to go on to college.

When I returned to Lubbock, a lot had changed on the music scene. I did not continue with that interest. Instead, I wanted to move on with my life. I was prepared to attend college, but the owners of the camera store had expanded their business into office copiers and printing equipment. They offered me a position as a sales service representative that required factory training for some of the new products. The pay was more than new college graduates were getting at the time. It required me to not enroll in college but instead go to New York City for training. I postponed college and accepted the position. I was in a hurry to grow up, so I married my girlfriend while she was still in high school. She finished high school the first year of our marriage.

My new job required me to travel during the week and call on newspapers and printing companies in small towns miles from Lubbock. Yes, there was alcohol in the mix. I would come home on the weekends, and again, would party with my new wife. Often joined by the owners of the camera store.

As I go down memory lane, I realize I must skip a lot of details to highlight the turning points as that camera store owner was fear that his behavior toward me would be revealed if I did not leave town.

Military school was a positive experience. However, many of the cadets were there, as they had also been sent there because they were out of control.

I was not in the official band company, but on one occasion, I sat in with a stage band that was an extension of the band company. This band played country music. I was invited to join the stage band, and because the counselors at Allen Academy were from Texas A&M University; we were allowed to play at some fraternity functions of the college. I was still able to enjoy playing music, but it was more structured, and the music was different. We did manage to find alcohol on some of those events, and I only got caught once. I was given a warning and never suffered any consequences.

Lubbock was a little too far from this school to go home on weekend leaves, so on several occasions I was allowed to go to Houston with some of my friends that lived there. We would party and consume alcohol during those times. In those years, marijuana was not part of the equation, and I was afraid of any drugs.

Military school was a positive experience for me. I managed to get my grades up and graduated from high school as a member of the National Honor Society. I was number thirteen in a graduating class of approximately 100 students. More importantly, I was able to go on to college.

When I returned to Lubbock, a lot had changed on the music scene. I did not continue with that interest. Instead, I wanted to move on with my life. I was prepared to attend college, but the owners of the camera store had expanded their business into office copiers and printing equipment. They offered me a position as a sales service representative that required factory training for some of the new products. The pay was more than new college graduates were getting at the time. It required me to not enroll in college but instead go to New York City for training. I postponed college and accepted the position. I was in a hurry to grow up, so I married my girlfriend while she was still in high school. She finished high school the first year of our marriage.

My new job required me to travel during the week and call on newspapers and printing companies in small towns miles from Lubbock. Yes, there was alcohol in the mix. I would come home on the weekends, and again, would party with my new wife. Often joined by the owners of the camera store.

As I go down memory lane, I realize I must skip a lot of details to highlight the turning points as they're related to my struggles with addiction and God's role in my life.

The point I need to make now is that by the time I was 28 years old, I had struggled with alcohol and had been introduced to marijuana. My life was in shambles. Now I know that even though I was not praying to God or serving him in any way, that he protected me many times for what might have happened. Even though I kept secrets of others' evil acts, I was able to resist the strong temptations before me from evil people with a strong influence in my life. More importantly, I realized how dangerous they were and managed to break away from their influence.

The Lubbock tornado of 1970 was the straw that broke the camel's back, as they say. Pressure from high debt, anger from my family, coupled with extreme damage to my print shop, led me to divorce. I sank deeper into the use of alcohol.

As I began to date after divorce, I reconnected with a girl that in high school had been homecoming queen and would never go out with me then. We became friends, and she was also addicted to alcohol. We started attending AA meetings together, and both got clean and sober. A former customer who was also a printer and member of AA had obtained an SBA loan to expand his business with modern technology. He employed me to help with his new venture and I worked as a salesperson for his company in Lubbock. Soon after we got his new business established, and I was sober, he convinced me to think the best thing for my future was to leave Lubbock. He wanted to open a sales office in Houston, Texas.

I moved to Houston, Texas on July 4th, 1972, to start a sales office for his company. The move from Lubbock, a city small enough that many people knew me and my family, to a large city like Houston, where nobody knew me, was quite an adjustment. I did not make a single sale for his company in the first month. I had obtained many new customers for him in Lubbock. He wanted to forget about the Houston office and have me return to Lubbock.

I did not want to do this. Houston was booming and jobs were plentiful. I decided to stay in Houston and contacted a placement agency, which sent me on four interviews almost immediately. In a few days, I got three job offers. The one I accepted was with the A. B. Dick Company. This was an old-line company involved in duplicating and printing equipment. They were a leader in this technology and highly respected during that time. I knew how to operate most of their equipment from my experience as a printer. I started as a sales representative for them in August 1972.

I was still sober and did not drink. This was awkward with my new job, as it involved socializing with peers and customers. Daily, they gathered at a popular happy hour spot and there were numerous trade shows. I was expected to attend all of these. They all served alcohol. I began to wonder if I could control my drinking, and eventually, as they say, fell off the wagon.

I had also met a young lady that was into smoking marijuana. I discovered that I could smoke marijuana and people would not detect it. So, I began smoking marijuana in private before I attended these events and was able to just drink slowly and control my drinking and joined in the activities. I stopped going to AA and my career advanced in an amazing way.

In a couple of years, I was promoted to sales manager in Los Angeles, California. I had been dating a sales secretary in the Houston office. We were married, and she moved to Los Angeles with me. We smoked marijuana together. In Los Angeles, we met some friends that also smoked marijuana. So, my pattern of not drinking much alcohol continued.

I stayed in Los Angeles for about 18 months (about 1 and a half years). I really enjoyed Los Angeles, but the cost of living there was much higher than Texas, so we moved back to Texas, and I was able to become a sales manager in the Houston Branch of A. B. Dick Company.

Soon after moving back, a business opportunity was presented to me to become co-owner of a printing supply company in Houston. The branch manager of the Houston branch of A.B. Dick was retiring, and a new manager was to take over his position. So, I left A.B. Dick and started working to build up this printing supply company.

It became apparent that my wife of four years and I were quite different when we were removed from the politics of the A. B. Dick Company. We divorced, and I continued as I single man working on my new venture.

This was at a time when inflation was rampant and the banks where we had large business loans raised interest rates tremendously. One day, without notice, they called our loans and emptied our bank account. My partner freaked out and disappeared. As it turned out, the bank only wanted to renegotiate our loan agreements, but this was not possible without his presence. So, the business closed, and the bank repossessed all the assets.

After a few months, the bank determined it was not easy to recover their loss with our specialized assets. The bank president told me that if I could sell those assets for enough to make a major contribution to the bank's loss after paying me a commission for selling them. He would not pursue a financial judgment against me. I accepted this offer and for about eighteen months; I worked as an agent for this bank.

During this time, I was really messed up. I slipped into some of my old habits and even experimented with other drugs such as cocaine and meth, not to mention the fact that alcohol was also a problem again. Somehow, I managed to sell enough assets to satisfy the bank, and I was able to become employed again with A. B. Dick Company.

I had met my current wife, who was also in an unpleasant situation. She had a small daughter and wanted to make a home for her. She had experienced a rough time before we met and together; we managed to create a healthy home life for her daughter. She was not addicted to drugs; in fact, she would not indulge in any drug abuse at all. Her only vice was that she liked her wine.

Our new lifestyle was to work hard all day and after our daughter went to bed, to relax, I would smoke my pot and she would have her glass of wine. Gradually, our lives began to improve, and we managed to start a business where we worked together. We are still together today. I can remember on one occasion where I lost control of myself using alcohol along with marijuana. After that, I lost my desire to drink at all, but continued to smoke marijuana.

When our daughter reached the age of 13, one day she came home telling us that she was going to get baptized at a new church nearby. One of her friends was a member there, and they were having a revival. I had never discussed God or religion with her, and she asked me if I knew anything about Jesus. When I replied, it was like I had a flashback to the time I had accepted Christ many years before. Then my response to her was that something that important could not happen without her mom and me being involved. So, we got dressed and went to the service as a family.

That event changed my life. I remember the sermon when the evangelist said that we are saved by faith and not by deeds, and that all that was necessary was a commitment to God through Jesus Christ. I could not contain myself and recommitted my life to Christ that day. I was, as they say, baptized by the Holy Spirit, a changed man. I still smoked marijuana, and I liked it.

I remember getting several translations of the Holy Bible and looking for information about smoking marijuana in the Bible. I was also praying to God for an answer. By this time, I knew that my smoking was a bad example for my children, and I had previously wanted to stop but just never could. I thought I could hide it from them, but really, that was not possible. I had always limited my offer and for about eighteen months; I worked as an agent for this bank.

During this time, I was really messed up. I slipped into some of my old habits and even experimented with other drugs such as cocaine and meth, not to mention the fact that alcohol was also a problem again. Somehow, I managed to sell enough assets to satisfy the bank, and I was able to become employed again with A. B. Dick Company.

I had met my current wife, who was also in an unpleasant situation. She had a small daughter and wanted to make a home for her. She had experienced a rough time before we met and together; we managed to create a healthy home life for her daughter. She was not addicted to drugs; in fact, she would not indulge in any drug abuse at all. Her only vice was that she liked her wine.

Our new lifestyle was to work hard all day and after our daughter went to bed, to relax, I would smoke my pot and she would have her glass of wine. Gradually, our lives began to improve, and we managed to start a business where we worked together. We are still together today. I can remember on one occasion where I lost control of myself using alcohol along with marijuana. After that, I lost my desire to drink at all, but continued to smoke marijuana.

When our daughter reached the age of 13, one day she came home telling us that she was going to get baptized at a new church nearby. One of her friends was a member there, and they were having a revival. I had never discussed God or religion with her, and she asked me if I knew anything about Jesus. When I replied, it was like I had a flashback to the time I had accepted Christ many years before. Then my response to her was that something that important could not happen without her mom and me being involved. So, we got dressed and went to the service as a family.

That event changed my life. I remember the sermon when the evangelist said that we are saved by faith and not by deeds, and that all that was necessary was a commitment to God through Jesus Christ. I could not contain myself and recommitted my life to Christ that day. I was, as they say, baptized by the Holy Spirit, a changed man. I still smoked marijuana, and I liked it.

I remember getting several translations of the Holy Bible and looking for information about smoking marijuana in the Bible. I was also praying to God for an answer. By this time, I knew that my smoking was a bad example for my children, and I had previously wanted to stop but just never could. I thought I could hide it from them, but really, that was not possible. I had always limited my procurement of marijuana to one person, and when that person would call, I would always give in.

One afternoon, God's answer to my prayers was almost audio-able and asked me if I really wanted to quit. When I said I did, he told me to flush what I had down the toilet. So as much as it hurt, I flushed an almost full bag of pot down the toilet. The miracle to me was the fact that the person that had called me for years to provide me with pot never called me again. So, after a period of withdrawal, I was once again free and clean of all the addictive substances.

As our family we became involved in church activities. I remained free from marijuana use for about five years. The church activities stopped after about three years because the churches in which we were involved seemed more interested in raising money for buildings than taking care of their members. In one, church leaders voted to remove the pastor. This pastor paid me a visit as he left town. He told me not to let the devil in churches spoil my relationship with God. He told me that whatever happened, going forward to maintain a strong relationship with God through prayer. Well, I can say that was the best advice I ever received.

My mom was getting older, had moved to Houston, and was living in an apartment of her own. My sister had also moved to Houston. When it became apparent that mom was going to need some assistance going forward. Her options were to move into an assisted living facility or live with one of her children. Before we realized that she also had Alzheimer's, we began construction of an addition to our house to accommodate her. She moved into our house with her own private apartment in the rear, and the plan was for my wife to be her caretaker.

The next life changing experience that confronted me was my wife was diagnosed with breast cancer. Her treatment involved surgery, which lasted 12 hours. That was the longest period that we never spoke in our relationship at the time. It was a tough time in my life. Mom at home with Alzheimer's and my wife recovering from cancer with treatments. Fortunately, by this time, our business, a courier service, was doing well, and our daughter was able to step in and help manage it.

The stress levels were high. One day, a customer came by our office and left me with a bag of pot. They said there was plenty of evidence that this could be helpful for cancer patients. Well, my wife wasn't interested, but I was, and I began smoking pot again. I must say the positive effects in my mind outweighed any negatives. At this point, I knew that pot gave a false since of well-being. I needed that. So, my pattern for use was simply to use it for a period, usually about a month, and then stop using it for about a month. I continued this pattern until I retired from the courier service around the year 2003.

Eventually my mom died, my wife recovered, and life returned to normal. Normal 12-hour days at the courier service working in a high-pressure environment. My wife and I would work hard, go home, and relax to get up and do it again the next day. I consumed my marijuana, and she consumed her wine before bed.

My prayer life continued but was not intense and really became just something I did. I guess you could say God was like the guy next door. We had a relationship, but I was not involved in his life, and he was not included 100% in mine. We spoke and respected each other, but nothing major occurred.

The Courier business was in a state of change. My personal efforts were directed at becoming a part of a network of same day delivery service companies that worked together to provide same day delivery nationwide using the airlines. The group was a network known as NextJet. We had a national advertising program that was getting customers. Our Houston operation was part of the service and had grown to the point that we had several deliveries each day. These were high priority, high-priced, profitable deliveries. The network allowed individual local operations to establish a sales effort on a national level with the

Internet. Our personal website was named 911couriers.com This was ready to go and introduced the same month as the World Trade Center bombings.

These bombings changed in a major way the practice of putting packages on an airline. Government regulations were put in place that it made our business model impossible to operate. I had worked on this project for about three years and this setback was frustrating.

I lost interest in the courier business and decided to pursue another direction as an occupation. My wife remained at our courier service, and we had some strategic partners who helped with overflow work. I left the courier business, although it still provided most of our income.

First, I got my real estate license and sold houses for about a year. During that time, I was exposed to karaoke. Since I had been interested in music in my younger days, this fascinated me. Also, technology was changing for karaoke.

I started a karaoke company and used my sales ability to establish karaoke shows in about 65 local bars and restaurants. I used the innovative technology to build karaoke systems, which I rented to host the shows. I also hosted shows myself.

Attending Karaoke shows involves using alcohol. I really had no desire to drink, and I think part of my decision to start a karaoke company and host shows was a way I could enjoy karaoke without having to participate in the drinking. I continued to smoke marijuana; in fact, my use of marijuana increased. I guess the fact that I came from an era when it was so dangerous to get caught with marijuana is the reason; I kept the actual smoking to myself. I usually smoke in private, but today, it has not been necessary to hide the fact that I smoke, even from doctors.

At first karaoke was just for fun. The idea of starting a karaoke company was really an interest in technology rather than thinking I would become a karaoke host. Interest in karaoke technology combined with my love for sales motivated me to start calling on bars to establish karaoke shows. I would find a venue, convince them to try karaoke, then I would find someone who I thought would make an excellent host and offer them some equipment to become a host. It was fun, and I was surprised and how many people could host a successful karaoke show.

I used direct mail in addition to making personal calls. One day, I got a response from the Wild West on Richmond. They already had karaoke but were looking to change host. I set up a demonstration to show them what we could provide. I had a host in mind, and he was going to show them what he could do. Well, he did not show up and there I was at the Wild West with equipment setup, and they were looking to see what we had to offer. So, I did the best I could to demonstrate the equipment. One of the primary features we had was that of computerized karaoke. We had a greater song selection. After the demonstration, or they might have called it an audition, I told them that the person I had in mind who did not show up would be a good fit at Wild West. He was a great entertainer himself and had a lot of experience in the entertainment industry. There were two ladies there; they looked at each other and smiled. They said we want you.

So, my first sincere effort to host a major show was at the Wild West. I must say, that was one of the greatest memories of karaoke hosting. It was on a Saturday night and their attendance at the Wild West on a Saturday evening was usually around 1000 people. It was primarily a dancing venue, and they had a live DJ in the wide area where the dance floor was. People would be lined up outside waiting to come in when people left. The capacity of the venue was about 600. The karaoke room was in the front of the building and closed off from the main area with a door. The idea for karaoke was to give people a place to take a break from dancing, so they wouldn't leave. Since the main dance floor had a DJ, they did not want a karaoke host that mind, and he was going to show them what he could do. Well, he did not show up and there I was at the Wild West with equipment setup, and they were looking to see what we had to offer. So, I did the best I could to demonstrate the equipment. One of the primary features we had was that of computerized karaoke. We had a greater song selection. After the demonstration, or they might have called it an audition, I told them that the person I had in mind who did not show up would be a good fit at Wild West. He was a great entertainer himself and had a lot of experience in the entertainment industry. There were two ladies there; they looked at each other and smiled. They said we want you.

So, my first sincere effort to host a major show was at the Wild West. I must say, that was one of the greatest memories of karaoke hosting. It was on a Saturday night and their attendance at the Wild West on a Saturday evening was usually around 1000 people. It was primarily a dancing venue, and they had a live DJ in the wide area where the dance floor was. People would be lined up outside waiting to come in when people left. The capacity of the venue was about 600. The karaoke room was in the front of the building and closed off from the main area with a door. The idea for karaoke was to give people a place to take a break from dancing, so they wouldn't leave. Since the main dance floor had a DJ, they did not want a karaoke host that

Attending Karaoke shows involves using alcohol. I really had no desire to drink, and I think part of my decision to start a karaoke company and host shows was a way I could enjoy karaoke without having to participate in the drinking. I continued to smoke marijuana; in fact, my use of marijuana increased. I guess the fact that I came from an era when it was so dangerous to get caught with marijuana is the reason; I kept the actual smoking to myself. I usually smoke in private, but today, it has not been necessary to hide the fact that I smoke, even from doctors.

At first karaoke was just for fun. The idea of starting a karaoke company was really an interest in technology rather than thinking I would become a karaoke host. Interest in karaoke technology combined with my love for sales motivated me to start calling on bars to establish karaoke shows. I would find a venue, convince them to try karaoke, then I would find someone who I thought would make an excellent host and offer them some equipment to become a host. It was fun, and I was surprised and how many people could host a successful karaoke show.

I used direct mail in addition to making personal calls. One day, I got a response from the Wild West on Richmond. They already had karaoke but were looking to change host. I set up a demonstration to show them what we could provide. I had a host in was also a DJ. So, when I did not have singers, I had to sing to keep the party going. This lasted about six years and over the years, many people would come to the Wild West, some of them only once or twice a year, and that is where I got to know so many of the people that I know today.

Eventually, a new aggressive karaoke company approached the Wild West home office, as they had around 15 locations statewide. They undercut my price. So, as they say, all good things must end. After a few months, Wild West discontinued karaoke altogether.

Most of my effort with a karaoke company was to establish new shows and put people in place to host them. Since I now had experience hosting busy shows, I would fill in for another host when they were unable to work. One skill I had was the ability to multitask, taking requests, searching for a song, and adjusting the sound efficiently. This was learned as a dispatcher for our courier service, but the advantage it gave me with karaoke was I could keep the music going without a filler or dead space. This enabled me to have more singers per hour than most hosts. So, my specialty became busy shows. After Wild West ended, the next busy show I was to host on a regular basis was Frankenstein's. They had two locations, and I worked at the Highway 6 location for about seven years and the Katy location until they closed after five years.

As with all new services and products, the rates got lower as the product or service became more established. This was true with karaoke hosting. As rates came down, there was less incentive to split the revenue between a rental and the actual hosting. So, I sold the systems to hosts that continued their own and stopped the practice of renting equipment to others.

I continued to host shows on my own. And it has been one of the most rewarding experiences of earning an income in my life. It started in 2003 and ended this past April in 2021. During this time, I have met so many wonderful people who have supported me as a host. I have hosted my own shows at Big John's, Coaches, Baker Street, Molly's, B. B. Wolf's, Nick's Jack's, Ashford Pub, and 510 Bar, to name a few. Working five nights per week.

On occasion, I would allow a customer or friend to buy me a shot. Tequila was my choice. However, I never wanted to drink to the point that I felt intoxicated. I recall recently someone making a comment on Facebook that they never saw me take a drink. In response, I made the statement that I drank a whole fifth of tequila, but it took me twelve years. While this was a joke, it is true.

The only chronic medical problem that I had was arthritis. Since they banned Celebrex, at times, I had severe knee pain and the only thing my doctor did was prescribe pain medication. This medication did not really help very much, and I never liked the side effects of pain medication. I soon learned that smoking marijuana gave me more relief than any pain medication, so my use of marijuana increased.

When I learned about CBD, immediately, I tried it and found more relief than any pain medication and better than with just marijuana. So, I did some research and eventually became a representative for a California company to sell their products. My main motivation to sell the product was to be able to buy it wholesale. I continued to sell it until the pandemic caused the company to cease operation. I continued to smoke marijuana daily, usually at night, one before my show and several after my show before going to bed.

I do still believe that CBD, in particular full spectrum CBD, has many health benefits as a food supplement if used in moderation. My experience with addiction to substance abuse has taught me that it is impossible to go from excessive use directly to moderation. One must first go through withdrawal of all the toxins in the body before they decide to return to moderation. At this point, I do not know what I will do as it relates to CBD or marijuana in the future.

When I get my checkups at the doctor, I continue too, always be healthy. That is a good thing, and I have attributed much of that to my use of food supplements and cannabis. However, conditions like my leg, fatigue and now dry eye caused me to wonder if I am experiencing side effects from its use. My dry eye was first diagnosed as an allergy to smoke and has now been proven to have no cause that can be identified. I have been tested for allergies, diabetes, immune disease, and anything else that normally causes dry eye. Unfortunately, doctors are not schooled in cannabis and cannot discuss concerns about cannabis with any confidence.

Recently, I have done more research on cannabis myself and discovered another symptom called CHS, which causes someone to vomit randomly. The research I have studied indicates that those with the condition go for days vomiting and it causes a serious condition. It has been determined to be a result of heavy or long-time use of cannabis. While I have not had the severe condition described in the research. I have on occasion vomited suddenly but managed to stop in a few minutes. I have always dismissed this, as perhaps I ate something.

Having a good understanding of how the endocannabinoid system works. I understand that today's medical system treats symptoms rather than causes. I believe it may be possible that too much cannabis can overload the endocannabinoid system. The only way to determine this I can see is to stop using cannabis. My hope is that first I will notice more energy, and that none of the conditions from arthritis will return, and that my dry eye will also go away. Only time will tell, and I expect it to take several months after I have withdrawn the toxins to repair my endocannabinoid system.

The purpose of this book is to help others who may have similar concerns to make decisions about cannabis use. There are many benefits, and like other medications, excess use may produce side effects. The only advice I can give anyone considering the use of CBD or marijuana is to use moderation. With dosage, start low and go slow with any increase.

As I write this, I am in my 7th week of withdrawal. I already have increased energy, do feel better, and have decided to lose a few pounds. I am not sure yet if my dry eye is gone; but I can tell you that my eyes are much clearer and feel better than in a long time. My leg is almost healed, and my teeth remain strong. Also, I see no evidence that my arthritis is returning. One of the claims of CBD is that not only does it relieve pain, but it also goes to work on the root cause. If it cured my arthritis, that alone would be amazing.

At 78 years old, I have been blessed. I feel God has been by my side since I first accepted Christ as a child. My prayer life and dependence on God have increased enormously in recent years and months. It's much easier to depend on God and have a relationship with him as we get older and less active. Regardless of your age or religion, I encourage you to be active in your prayer life with God. Also, take the time to meditate and listen to his voice. I believe that God's will for every one of us is to have a personal relationship. In doing so, he can guide you to do what is right and will protect you from the temptation of the devil. God wants you to have free choice and will provide you with options that will glorify Him.

Chapter Nine

Conclusion

When I first told a few of my friends that I had decided to stop smoking marijuana, the first question was why? I thought, well, it would take a book to answer that question. So, I have authored a book.

The message I hope I portray is not one that says I am 100% for or against marijuana. But rather, I feel, it is time for more research and legalization. Cannabis was mainstream before the United States was even an idea. Our founders, including George Washington and others, were hemp farmers. The original constitution was written on hemp paper. The first Bible was printed on hemp paper. Even early industrialists like Henry Ford were also hemp farmers. In 1943 Ford built a prototype of an automobile that was almost 100% made from hemp and used hemp biofuels to power it.

At the turn of the 20th century. Evil began to take control of our government. Amendments have been made to our constitution that have caused us to stray from the original guidelines for America. Industrialists greedy for profit, have taken control of our government, laws, and restrictions put in place under the pretense of protecting us. When they were protecting greedy special interest. Cannabis is just one of the issues we have been lied about by our government.

We have broken the 75-year prohibition of cannabis, but we have not yet restored all the benefits it may provide humanity. That will take time. Our country has grown and now is managed by bureaucracy and self-serving leadership. This leadership tells us what they want us to believe to advance their own agenda. Cannabis could go a long way to improving concerns over climate change, but this fact is being ignored by politicians.

Our only protection against misguided information is from God. The only way we will find peace on earth is with God. I believe the spirit within each one of us is, in fact, the image of God. We are all his children. We can establish a meaningful relationship with our father through prayer. That prayer must come from deep in our hearts. What God wants from each of us is that personal relationship where we include him in everything we do and follow his direction to satisfy our own hearts.

Cannabis is just one issue that we have allowed evil to obstruct. I have stopped using cannabis and marijuana because I feel I may have used it in excess. God tells us that everything on this earth is here for the greater good, but also says moderation should be used in all things. I have experienced other addictions, and I believe no one must stop entirely to restore your body. If I return to the use of cannabis in the future, I know I will practice moderation.

I smoked marijuana for many years without problems by using a pattern of moderation. The overuse came when I started using CBD with it; I feel. I simply took too much and overloaded my cannabinol system.

I hope I have been able to provide a better understanding of cannabis with this book. Thank you for reading it and I would like to invite you to join my Facebook page if you have not already. We can interact there in real time. My Facebook page is under my name, Vern Kirby. May God bless you.

www.ingramcontent.com/pod-product-compliance
Lightning Source LLC
Chambersburg PA
CBHW050245220526
45465CB00002B/552